The Complete REBT
Whether you're learnin[g Rational Emotive Behavior]
Therapy (REBT) to wo[rk on yourself or learning how to]
use it, this program benefits everyone. Comprised of nine booklets, videos, and workbooks, plus an audiocassette album, this program helps every kind of learner through print, sight, and sound.

For the learner . . .
Learn by reading: REBT booklets
- introduce you to the *ABC*'s of REBT
- help you understand your past actions and how you can turn them around

Learn by seeing and hearing: REBT videos and audiocassettes
- see yourself through others—in real-life situations
- review the videos and audios whenever and wherever you want

Learn by doing: REBT workbooks
- test yourself on the workbooks' questions
- practice and develop the skill of using REBT in your everyday life

For the clinician . . .
A cognitive approach: REBT booklets
- begin the phase of defining the problem
- meet your educational needs for both individual and group sessions

An emotive response: REBT videos and audiocassettes
- provide dramatic vignettes and graphic reminders that reinforce core REBT principles
- facilitate group communication, promoting peer-to-peer learning

A behavioral technique: REBT workbooks
- function as effective assessment and evaluation tools
- provide step-by-step guidelines for client goal-setting and goal achievement

For price and order information, or a free catalog, please call our Telephone Representatives.

HAZELDEN
1-800-328-9000 (Toll-Free U.S. and Canada)
1-651-213-4000 (Outside the U.S. and Canada)
1-651-213-4590 (24-Hour Fax)
www.hazelden.org (World Wide Web on the Internet)

15251 Pleasant Valley Road • P.O. Box 176
Center City, MN 55012-0176

The following titles compose the complete REBT learning program. Each is available in booklet, workbook, audio, and video format:

*Understanding • Anger • Perfectionism
Anxiety and Worry • Depression • Shame
Grief • Guilt • Self-Esteem*

Rational Emotive Behavior Therapy

Depression
Revised
Tim Sheehan, Ph.D.

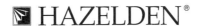

Hazelden
Center City, Minnesota 55012-0176

©1990, 1992, 2002 by Hazelden Foundation
All rights reserved. Published 1990
Second edition 1992
Third edition 2002
Printed in the United States of America
No portion of this publication may be reproduced in any manner without the written permission of the publisher

ISBN: 1-56838-957-4

The stories in this booklet are composites of many individuals. Any similarity to any one person is purely coincidental.

About the booklet
This booklet explains the three main types of depression, their origins, and how working through depression with Rational Emotive Behavior Therapy (REBT) can help us reduce the risk of relapse. This booklet is based on the work of Dr. Albert Ellis and his Rational Emotive Behavior Therapy.

Dr. Ellis, who first articulated Rational-Emotive Therapy (RET) in the 1950s, changed the name in the 1990s to Rational Emotive Behavior Therapy (REBT) to more accurately reflect the role behavior plays in gauging changes in thinking. While the therapeutic approach remains the same, the pamphlets, workbooks, audios, and videos in this series have been changed to reflect the updated name.

About the author
Timothy J. Sheehan, Ph.D., is Vice President, Academic Affairs, for the Hazelden Foundation's Education Division.

Dr. Sheehan holds a Doctorate Degree in Clinical Psychology and has held numerous positions over the past twenty years at Hazelden, including leadership roles in clinical psychology and health care services, as well as administrative roles in adult, youth, and transitional care. He is the author of a sequence of pamphlets and workbooks addressing the application of Rational Emotive Behavior Therapy for depression and shame as well as *Facing an Eating Disorder in Recovery* and *Freedom from Compulsion: An Eating Disorder Workbook*. He is also the author of "The Disease Model" in McCrady and Epstein's *Addictions: A Comprehensive Guidebook*. He is a professor in Hazelden's Graduate School in Addiction Studies and an adjunct associate professor in the graduate school of psychology at St. Mary's University of Minnesota.

Introduction

Happiness is a personal sense of well-being; it's having the capacity to feel joy, contentment, and fulfillment. Happiness is one of the most basic motivators of human behavior. Most people strive to be happy. Even the Declaration of Independence refers to the "pursuit of happiness" as a basic human right. For those of us recovering from an addictive behavior, happiness is something we hope to build into our recovery.

Happiness and sadness are not opposite sides of the same coin. In some situations, we might feel both happy and sad. For instance, in chemical dependency treatment we might feel happy that we are not being self-destructive but sad because we are no longer getting high.

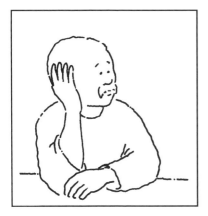

Sadness is part of life—it's an emotion that signals to us that something has been changed or lost. Everyone feels sad at one time or another. For most of us, sadness is temporary. As we shed our tears, our sadness ebbs. Our capacity for happiness continues.

Most of us equate *depression* with uncomfortable feelings such as sadness or grief. Depression, however, is more than a feeling. While sadness may be a symptom of depression, most depression also involves self-defeating thoughts, feelings, and behaviors that limit our capacity for joy, impair our ability to be responsible, and isolate us from others.

The *ABC* process described in this booklet is based on the work of Dr. Albert Ellis and his Rational Emotive Behavior Therapy.

Depression varies in intensity. Some depression is mild and has only a minimal impact on a person's life. Other depression is more severe, resulting in sleep loss, appetite changes, fatigue, feelings of gloom, and even thoughts of suicide.

Depression—it's not all the same
For most of us, feelings of depression can stem from a number of sources, including:
1. loss or change;
2. changes or imbalances in brain chemistry;
3. self-defeating belief systems.

In fact, many of us feel depressed as a result of elements stemming from all three.

Nursing the wounds left by change and loss
Feelings of sadness and depression are often related to prolonged grief; that is, they usually happen as the result of a loss. Grief is a natural reaction that helps us accept changes and losses in life. Losing a loved one, losing a job, becoming physically disabled, or moving away from a familiar place can all cause grief. Grief may occur in stages, often starting with disbelief or denial, then sadness, and then acceptance of the loss. Sometimes we may feel angry over a loss or even with a loved one for leaving or dying.

Treatment. By understanding and expressing our feelings, we can let the grieving process heal the wounds left by the change and losses in our lives. As time goes on, we get better at recognizing and dealing with reactive depression. Healthy grief is accompanied by unhealthy depression when we demand that serious losses must not and should not happen, and insist that we can't ever be happy when they do. We may also think that life is not worth living because of them.

Sometimes it's not a matter of loss
In contrast to prolonged grief, some depression seems to have little relation to stressors or losses in our lives. We find ourselves feeling gradually unhappy and listless. There is little joy in our lives. We may sleep too much or find ourselves tired and unable to sleep. Feelings of depression can be related to changes or imbalances in our brain chemistry. For some of us, there seems to be a strong genetic link. We have family histories of depression. In fact, some of us may have been born with a biological predisposition to feel depressed easily. Chemical imbalances are thought to trigger a number of symptoms of depression, including:
- feelings of melancholy
- reduced ability to feel pleasure
- loss of interest in others
- reduced sexual drives

Changes in sleep and appetite patterns are common with severe depression. A person suffering from severe depression might sleep too much, yet feel tired. Or he or she might sleep fitfully or not at all. Appetite may also be affected. Feelings of hunger become distorted and a person may either eat much less or more than usual.

Treatment. Antidepressant medication, in addition to counseling and therapy, is often used to treat severe depression. Antidepressants help to counteract the biochemical imbalance by stimulating the production of brain chemicals that are lacking or by helping the brain burn up chemicals that are overabundant. Antidepressant medication can be used in chemical dependency recovery because it is not mood-altering; instead, it diminishes the symptoms associated with depression.

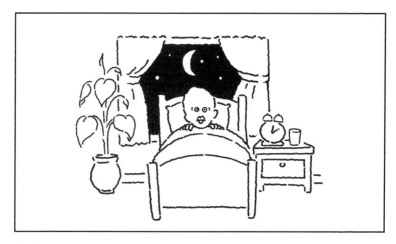

Sue's story
For more than two years, Sue, a nurse, had been free from symptoms of bulimia. She had struggled with binge eating since her late teens. With the help of her therapist and group, Sue had been able to change her behavior. Because Sue had been doing so well, she didn't understand the changes that had begun to happen recently. She was waking up early, as early as 3:00 A.M., and wasn't able to get back to sleep. Though she stuck to her meal plan, she wasn't hungry when she ate. Sue was also constantly tired, and she couldn't concentrate at work. Sue was becoming depressed. She couldn't think clearly and began overreacting to some situations. Gradually, Sue's feelings of helplessness and hopelessness deepened.

A nurse at heart, Sue sought medical attention. Following a thorough physical examination, her internist arranged for Sue to see a psychiatrist. The psychiatrist diagnosed Sue's symptoms as being the result of severe depression and recommended antidepressant medication in addition to individual therapy. She knew from nursing school that antidepressants were not addictive. She also knew that it would be at least two weeks before she benefited from the medication and that there might be some side effects but that they would last only a short time.

Sue's sleeping pattern eventually returned to normal, her appetite came back, and she no longer felt helpless and hopeless. She found it much easier to deal with upsetting situations at work and in her personal life. The medication had not left her euphoric or high—it had simply restored her to her normal state.

Like most people treated with antidepressant medication, Sue regularly saw her psychiatrist, who evaluated her symptoms and determined when to reduce and discontinue the medication. Within twelve months, Sue was medication-free. Her psychiatrist explained to her that most people who suffer from depression respond positively to medication. They successfully learn to change self-defeating belief systems and have a low rate of relapse back to depression once medication is discontinued. For some people, depression is more chronic and medication is used for a longer time. A small number of people may need antidepressants and medication for as long as they live.

Some call it stinkin' thinkin'
Our character is made up of the attitudes that shape our behavior, which includes how we form and maintain relationships, stay true to our values, balance ourselves emotionally, and cope with stress. Character develops slowly and with practice and is a sign of maturity.

For most of us with an addictive illness and emotional problems, the natural process of character development has been delayed. We have not had as much practice as we need to become mature. Consequently, our attitudes may be less than mature. As a result, we make unrealistic demands on ourselves, anticipate the worst from others, exaggerate routine problems, and eventually undermine our own self-worth.

Our attitudes actually prevent us from attaining our desired goal of a happier, more fulfilling life. Attitudes that are less than mature keep us from having fulfilling relationships, undermine our values, lessen our ability to cope with stress, and rob us of happiness. Self-defeating attitudes and emotional immaturity frequently lead to feelings of depression.

All types of depression—mild, moderate, and severe—are associated with deeply held negative beliefs about ourselves that lead us to say things such as, "My relationships are awful and I can't possibly cope any longer," and "I am totally unlovable." Because depression is linked to our belief system, changing our thinking is a key to recovery and staving off future problems with depression. Severe, moderate, or mild depressions all show improvement as we learn to understand our feelings and how our attitudes and behaviors can be used to help reduce or eliminate persistent feelings of depression.

Treatment. All types of depression, mild, moderate, and severe, can be eased with self-help—by changing our self-defeating attitudes, for instance, so we can cope with our feelings more effectively. Individual counseling or therapy that helps us understand and practice new attitudes and behaviors is instrumental for many of us to challenge deeply held beliefs and old behavior patterns that defeat our goal of living a happier life. Because depression robs us of our serenity, it can easily trigger a relapse to self-defeating behavior patterns, including a return to addictive behaviors.

Here is a brief review of the three major sources of depression. The first type, *prolonged grief*,
- acts in response to stress, such as the loss of a loved one
- is often associated with the dogmatic demand that a serious loss must not exist
- is resolved in stages
- causes temporary interruption of day-to-day functioning

The second type, *severe depression*,
- is often characterized by physical symptoms, particularly disrupted sleeping and eating patterns. The symptoms tend to be severe, often interrupting work and social functioning
- is associated with chemical imbalances in the brain
- may be found more frequently in alcoholics and family members of alcoholics
- is commonly associated with a family history of depression
- is characterized by deeply held, self-defeating belief systems.

The third type, *mild to moderate depression*,
- is typically determined by deeply ingrained patterns of thinking
- stems from emotional immaturity associated with addiction
- is often due to self-defeating behaviors that increase feelings of hopelessness and despair
- acts as a block to a contented recovery and tends to be recurrent unless treated properly.

Belief systems
Regardless of what type of depression we suffer from, our belief system plays a vital role in maintaining and intensifying depression.

Our belief system is made up of the thoughts and attitudes that help us give meaning to the events in our life.

We use our belief system to evaluate and judge situations and ourselves. Belief systems that trigger feelings of depression often involve self-downing. Self-downing beliefs lead us to see our future in the worst possible light, interpret our situation as hopeless, and make us feel worthless. But we can change our self-downing beliefs. We have a choice about what we believe. When we change our self-downing beliefs, we can diffuse our depression.

Jim's story
Jim had been a rowdy adolescent. His father, an active alcoholic, was rarely involved in Jim's life during his youth. Jim's mother was a truly unhappy woman who often withdrew from the rest of the family, perhaps in an attempt to quiet her own turmoil. This left Jim without the love and guidance he needed. Consequently, Jim's childhood was characterized by a lack of self-discipline and by the pursuit of instant gratification and cheap thrills. He remained much the same as he entered adulthood.

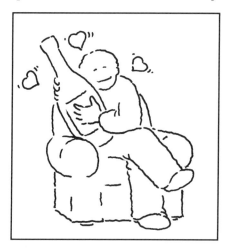

Drinking came early and easily for Jim. "Love in a bottle," he called it. It seemed to give Jim the joy and fulfillment his life lacked. Eventually, however, his drinking became a problem. A severe alcoholic by his early twenties, Jim ended up in a treatment center. After treatment, Jim began to learn how to live his life without drinking. It wasn't easy, but he went to Alcoholics Anonymous (AA) meetings every week and tried to work his recovery program. Nonetheless, Jim soon realized that all of his problems didn't go away when he stopped drinking. He recalled having been told while in treatment that he suffered from a personality disorder—deeply ingrained character traits that could make ongoing behavior change difficult. He struggled with staying sober through periods of despair and hopelessness. Sometimes it was hard for him to believe that he could be restored to a sane, healthy life.

When things went wrong, Jim was easily distraught and ready to throw in the towel. To him, life seemed too hard to keep trying. Even small disappointments depressed him.

Jim had problems finding a lasting relationship and couldn't concentrate on his work. He learned that he had not been chosen for a supervisory position he had applied for. The world around him seemed forbidding and overwhelming. Jim viewed his future in a pessimistic light. He blamed his job and "bad breaks" for his depression.

Because of his depression, Jim became more unproductive at work. And he didn't often feel like being around other people. Instead, he would stay in his room for hours at a time, miss a day of work, skip an AA meeting, or cancel a social engagement. Although his attempts to lick his wounds were meant as a remedy, Jim's isolation only deepened his depression. He had even *more* time to dwell on the misfortunes in his life.

Jim's episodes of depression were short-lived, usually lasting from a few hours to a few days. While he did think of drinking to solve his feelings of hopelessness and helplessness, he didn't consider suicide. Jim's depression kept him from getting to sleep as soon as he liked, though he rarely had significant sleep problems.

What Jim didn't realize was that his depression wasn't caused by the events in his life. After all, many people have managed to stay optimistic even in the face of discouraging events. Jim's depression was more the result of his belief system and his interpretations of his experiences than of actual events.

Using REBT to work through gloom and doom

Let's use a self-help approach called Rational Emotive Behavior Therapy (REBT) to take a closer look at the relationship between our thoughts and feelings. We'll use Jim's story as an example. REBT, developed by Dr. Albert Ellis, says that when an event happens, we interpret it based on our thoughts and beliefs. This interpretation triggers our emotional response. Our interpretation of events can be negative, neutral, or positive. The more negative our interpretation of events, and the more we insist that negative event absolutely *must* not exist, the more depressed we are likely to feel.

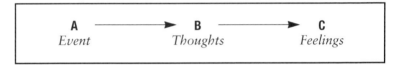

For example, the more Jim viewed himself as helpless, the more he reinforced his feelings of despair. The more he interpreted his environment as overwhelming, the more his depression deepened. The more he looked at his future through dark-colored glasses, the more hopeless he felt.

Feelings of depression and self-defeating thoughts and behavior go hand in hand. Jim's depression not only caused him to feel poorly, it also contributed to his self-defeating ways. When we're depressed, self-defeating behavior may sometimes look like a good, or even the only, solution, but it actually makes our problems worse. For example, Jim's withdrawal and inability to concentrate on his work made

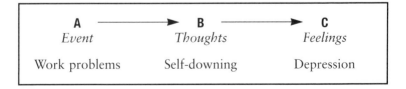

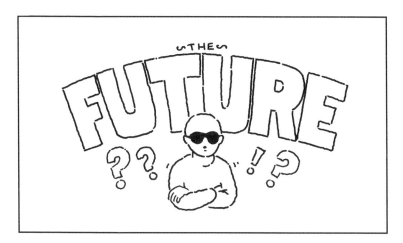

his depression worse. Remember, self-defeating behavior may dull pain, but it does not eliminate pain or solve the problem of depression.

With depression, the resulting behavior often involves a quick fix—a behavior that seems to dull the pain. But in reality, the behavior does not solve the problem. Whenever we feel a strong emotion, a behavioral urge comes along with it. In Jim's case, the urge to pull away from others was linked to his depression. A self-destructive cycle followed. It began with an unpleasant or unfortunate event (A), followed by negative, self-downing thoughts (B), which resulted in feelings of depression (C). Jim's self-defeating behavior reinforced his feelings of hopelessness and perpetuated his depression. Also, when we observe our depression and make it into a new or secondary problem (A) and tell ourselves, "I must not be depressed! I'm no good for being depressed!" (B) we get depressed about our depression (C)—and thereby make ourselves doubly depressed.

Changing our thinking
If Jim were to change his negative interpretations to more neutral or objective interpretations, his feelings would also change. He would feel less depressed. But to change his thinking, Jim needs to confront the way he views his experiences.

Self-downing attitudes are part of a negative belief system. A negative belief system is made up of both *unrealistic demands* and *negative exaggerations*. An example of an unrealistic demand is the belief that we should have absolute control over our situations, feelings, and other people's behavior. We may also harbor unrealistic demands for self-fulfillment or gratification. Negative exaggerations portray merely unfortunate or inconvenient incidents as catastrophic events. Both negative exaggerations and unrealistic demands stem from our character defects. Remember, if we have been burdened by long-term emotional problems and an addictive illness, we haven't had the practice we need to become mature.

Jim entered the world of work with a fair amount of adolescent idealism. He believed that he *should* be, *had* to be, the best employee; *had* to outperform his colleagues; and *had* to gain a quick promotion. His beliefs were full of unrealistic demands. When Jim's demands weren't realized, he exaggerated his misfortune, turning disappointment into devastation.

Tips for breaking the cycle of depression
In order to break the self-defeating cycle of depression, here are a few helpful tips:
- Stop focusing on the situation or event.
- Accept your feelings.
- Aim for more appropriate feelings, such as sadness, disappointment, and frustration, instead of depression and despair.

- Take inventory of your belief system. Look out for unrealistic demands and negative exaggerations.
- Question your logic. Replace self-downing logic with more objective logic.

Questioning our logic is like having a debate with ourselves. It begins an internal discussion that helps us to break up irrational beliefs and to view our situations more objectively. By questioning our logic, we put on the brakes and think before taking action. One of the ways to question our logic is to ask ourselves the following questions:
- Who said it must be so?
- What is the evidence?
- Where is the proof?
- Is this fact or opinion?

After we question our logic, we can establish a realistic goal and consider the many consequences of our reaction to a situation, including our physical and mental health. Asking ourselves, *What would I like to have happen?* will help us set our goal. For most of us, our first priority is to protect the gains we've already made. We would prefer to live productive, healthy lives with as little depression as possible. We might develop a goal that reads something like this: *To continue making behavior changes while learning to reduce my feelings of depression.*

We're not quite finished yet. The last phase is crucial—we also need to figure out *how* we are going to reach our goal. What constructive action can we take that will help us reach our goal? By making a list of specific actions, we create a plan that will help us achieve it.

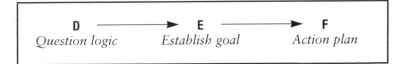

More about Jim
Let's put it all together in an example. We'll continue with Jim's story.

Having been passed over for a recent promotion, Jim sank into depression. Fortunately, he had been introduced to REBT while he was in treatment for alcoholism. So, after feeling depressed for a while, rather than blaming his work situation, Jim took an inventory of his belief system. He decided to outline his belief system on paper so he could see his ideas more clearly. First, Jim identified the event (A): not being chosen for the supervisory position. In describing the event, Jim wrote only the facts of the situation, not his opinion of it.

Next, Jim identified his thoughts (B), including unrealistic demands and negative exaggerations. He listed each thought one by one:
 1. I must not fail or get rejected.
 2. I can't do anything right.
 3. I'm doomed to an awful future.
 4. No one will ever give me a break.

Since Jim had already recognized his self-defeating pattern of withdrawal caused by his feelings of depression (C), he went on to question his logic (D) to reduce his feelings of depression and to avoid isolating himself. Here are some of the questions and statements Jim used to challenge his logic:
 1. Why must I never fail or get rejected?
 2. What evidence do I have that I've never done anything right?

3. What proof do I have that I'm doomed to an awful future? Is this fact or opinion?
4. Who says no one will ever give me a break?
5. True, it's disappointing not to get the promotion, but it's certainly not the end of the world.
6. Stop "catastrophizing"!

As Jim questioned each belief, he felt less depressed but still somewhat disappointed. Jim felt, though, that he could deal much more easily with the appropriate feeling of disappointment than with the feeling of depression. *After all, who wouldn't be disappointed after missing a promotion?* he said to himself. As a result, he set a goal (E) to help guide his future actions. Jim understood that his tendency to isolate himself put him in danger of relapsing to his pattern of self-defeating behavior. He did not want to repeat past mistakes, such as canceling social engagements or spending hours alone in his room. These didn't seem like positive choices anymore. He preferred to be happy and to avoid feeling depressed. Jim wrote out his goal: "To feel happy more often in the future." Next, Jim brainstormed the actions (F) he could take to reach his goal. His list was simple and practical:

- To schedule some activities with friends in the near future so I don't isolate myself.
- To get together with a close friend or family member and talk about my disappointment in not getting the job so my loved ones know I'm in need of support.
- To take constructive action in talking to my boss about why I didn't get the promotion—perhaps it has nothing to do with my performance. If it does, perhaps I disagree with my boss about my ability to do the job.

Jim realized that this was a good start. Rather than

focusing on his unfortunate situation or blaming his supervisor at work, Jim began to accept responsibility for his own well-being. He felt less victimized by his feelings and more empowered to take constructive action.

Carol's story
Carol was relieved. The antidepressant medication had eased her sleepless nights, profound feelings of gloom, and appetite loss. Carol remembered how her mother had suffered from depression when Carol was an adolescent. Carol was recovering from a dependency on painkillers and minor tranquilizers. A Narcotics Anonymous member for years, Carol worried about the potential of relapse now that she was taking medication. She wondered, *Does the use of medication reflect poorly on how I work my program? Should I continue with my Twelve Step program? Will antidepressant medication lead me back to other pills?*

Conscientious about her well-being, Carol consulted both a psychiatrist who was knowledgeable about addiction and a psychologist who specialized in treating dual disorders. Assured that antidepressant medication was safe for her, Carol was told to continue with the prescribed dose and report any unusual side effects. Carol learned that for many people, depression is linked to relapse. She told herself that taking the antidepressant medication was helpful to her recovery because it reduced her fatigue and depression.

Nonetheless, Carol continued to have difficulty accepting that she needed medication. She remembered how she had used REBT to challenge feelings of despair and self-pity in early recovery, but now her task was different. Now more than ever she needed to learn self-help methods to ease her depression and accept the recommendation for medication. She wondered if REBT might help.

Carol learned that the answer was yes. Even in cases of

severe depression, challenging our belief system plays an important role in reducing our stress and bolstering our ability to cope. For many people, both antidepressant medication and REBT are helpful in responding to severe depression. In fact, the continued use of REBT even when antidepressant medication is no longer needed can help prevent further depression.

Reflecting, Carol realized that she was powerless over her depression. *If I had been able to will my depression away, I would have by now,* she thought. Bolstered by her recollection of the behaviors she had already changed in recovery from her addiction, Carol felt more hopeful. Taking action, Carol took an inventory of her beliefs, watching out for unrealistic demands and negative exaggerations. She also wrote about the beliefs and feelings that made it difficult for her to take the antidepressant medication.

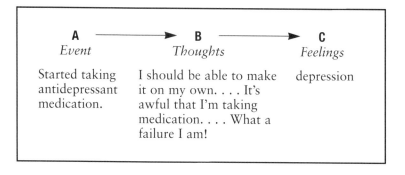

Next, Carol began to question her logic (*D*). As she looked more closely at her thinking, Carol felt less saddened, which helped her set a goal (*E*). Then she developed an action plan (*F*).

D →	E →	F
Question logic	*Establish goal*	*Action plan*
Who says I should be making it on my own? Aren't serenity and recovery also about trusting others? . . . What evidence do I have that taking an antidepressant is awful? . . . Who says I'm a failure? Where is the proof that I'm a failure? . . . My years of abstinence suggest that I must be doing something right. . . . Stop feeling sorry for yourself.	To continue my recovery while accepting that I may need help to deal with my depression	Initiate participation in a dual disorder support group. . . . Maintain contact with NA. . . . Maintain appointments with psychiatrist to evaluate my symptoms. . . . Reduce medication within next nine months. . . . Report unusual side effects.

Later, Carol shared her action plan with her psychologist. While impressed with Carol's efforts, her psychiatrist wondered if Carol had fully addressed the acceptance issue. Carol had recognized her need for professional help, but her psychologist wondered if Carol had accepted her depression was part of a dual disorder—a mental health problem as serious as her addiction. Looking more closely, Carol wrote her thoughts (*B*). This time she focused only on her thoughts about her depression.

B Thoughts	C Feelings	D Question logic
I should have known better than to let myself get so depressed.	sadness	Who says I should have known better?
It's awful to suffer from depression. I hate myself for allowing it.	sadness	Who says humans must always feel happy? Of course it's no fun being depressed, but with REBT and my medication I feel okay.
It's all so unfair; everyone is happy in recovery but me.	sadness	Who says life is always fair? I'm happy I can get help.

Carol was surprised to find such an obvious pattern of unrealistic demands. She acknowledged her feelings of sadness (C), and then questioned her logic (D) automatically.

As Carol talked further with her psychologist, she recognized that she needed to accept both her medication and her depression. Carol was able to do this because she understood her severe depression as an illness that coexisted with her addiction.

Consequently, Carol added the following items to her action plan (F):
- Attack self-downing beliefs with daily affirmations, such as *I'm Carol, a worthwhile, fallible woman. I'm doing the best I can, and I'm grateful for what I have accomplished.*
- Continue to take inventory of my beliefs, watching out for unrealistic demands and negative exaggerations.

Important points to remember

1. REBT is a therapy as well as a self-help method. REBT focuses on personal choice, empowerment, and everyone's ability to cope with feelings such as depression without resorting to self-defeating behaviors.

2. Depression is more than just an emotion. There are three basic sources of depression—stressors in our lives, such as change or loss; changes or imbalances in our brain chemistry; and deeply held, self-defeating belief systems. Depression has been consistently associated with relapse to addictive behaviors.

3. Grief is a psychological process involving feelings of depression that unfold when we experience a change or loss, such as losing a job or a loved one. Grief is resolved with time and emotional support, but especially by viewing losses as unfortunate and temporarily handicapping, not as catastrophic.

4. *Severe depression* is often characterized by physical symptoms that occur over a period of two or three weeks and often include sleep problems or appetite changes. For most people, following a Twelve Step program, using REBT, and taking antidepressant medication are the best ways to reduce symptoms of depression, to prevent relapse to addictive behaviors, and to stave off future problems with depression.

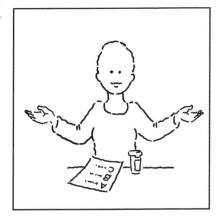

5. *Mild to moderate depression* is most commonly associated with early recovery from chemical dependency and is usually triggered by unrealistic demands we make on ourselves or our negative exaggeration of events. These demands are frequently a part of a self-downing belief system. This type of depression usually includes feelings of despair and hopelessness and tends to be relatively short-lived, but it can be recurrent if it is not treated properly.

6. REBT is particularly helpful in coping with depression because it can reduce the feelings of despair and hopelessness that may trigger relapse. Regular use of REBT will help you reduce emotional upset and develop behaviors that will help you reach your goals.

7. Don't hesitate to ask for help. Resources to help you through depression include your physician, psychologist, social worker, chemical dependency counselor, or psychiatrist. Make sure the resource you choose has a working knowledge of both addiction and psychological disorders.

Practice doesn't make perfect, but it sure helps
REBT is only helpful if it is applied. While the principles of REBT are simple, applying them is sometimes difficult. The only way to make REBT easy is through practice. For many of us, our belief systems are deeply ingrained. Only by challenging our logic daily can we become more objective about our attitudes.

To make REBT a part of your recovery, here are a few simple steps. Begin with an easy example. Don't start with the biggest disappointment of your life. You need success with simpler, easier problems before you tackle the more difficult ones.

1. Start by identifying upset feelings (C).

2. List your thoughts (B). Pay special attention to unrealistic demands and negative exaggerations. Remember, when you feel depressed, your belief system is apt to include some self-downing beliefs.

3. Describe the event (A). Try to be objective; stick to the facts.

4. Question your logic (D). This is the hard part. Have a debate with yourself. Challenge your thinking. Many people begin by asking themselves such questions as *Who said it must be so? What is the evidence? What is the proof? Is this fact or opinion?*

5. Identify your goal (E). Here, you want to discover what you would like to have happen. Remember, your goals need to include an emotional component, such as feeling less depressed or gaining hope.

6. Develop an action plan (F). You can do this by brainstorming all of the constructive actions you could take to realize your goal. You might want to reread the stories in this pamphlet for some more ideas. Remember, an action plan lists all of the behaviors you can take to reach your goal.

There is no time like the present.

Hazelden Publishing and Educational Services is a division of the Hazelden Foundation, a not-for-profit organization. Since 1949, Hazelden has been a leader in promoting the dignity and treatment of people afflicted with the disease of chemical dependency.

The mission of the foundation is to improve the quality of life for individuals, families, and communities by providing a national continuum of information, education, and recovery services that are widely accessible; to advance the field through research and training; and to improve our quality and effectiveness through continuous improvement and innovation.

Stemming from that, the mission of this division is to provide quality information and support to people wherever they may be in their personal journey—from education and early intervention, through treatment and recovery, to personal and spiritual growth.

Although our treatment programs do not necessarily use everything Hazelden publishes, our bibliotherapeutic materials support our mission and the Twelve Step philosophy upon which it is based. We encourage your comments and feedback.

The headquarters of the Hazelden Foundation are in Center City, Minnesota. Additional treatment facilities are located in Chicago, Illinois; New York, New York; Plymouth, Minnesota; St. Paul, Minnesota; and West Palm Beach, Florida. At these sites, we provide a continuum of care for men and women of all ages. Our Plymouth facility is designed specifically for youth and families.

For more information on Hazelden, please call **1-800-257-7800**. Or you may access our World Wide Web site on the Internet at **www.hazelden.org**.